ESTABLISHING A CAREER IN SPORTS MEDICINE

Plan Your Career In Sports Medicine Now And Enjoy The Many Possibilities For Personal Advancement It Offers

D1472548

Sports & Fitness

Sports medicine is a sub specialty of the medical field that is somewhat confusing to some people. Because of the fact that sports is not medicine, it is a bit of a misleading term, however, the term is intended to represent the doctors and other medical staff who are in the practice of treating and diagnosing athletes and sports related injuries. The professionals who are actively involved in the sports medicine field ranges from standard doctors, physical therapists, surgeons, and even athletic trainers and other similar careers.

Are you considering a career in the field of sports medicine? Let this comprehensive career guidebook assist you in your contemplation, planning for your education and training, and setting up your career path. Inside this book you will discover:

- A short description of sports medicine, including a brief historical account
- A guide for self-assessment to help you examine if this is the right career choice for you
- Career possibilities and job opportunities

The field of sports medicine is vast and there are a lot of opportunities that can be made. As in all areas of life, planning and goal-setting is key. Plan for your career in sports medicine now and get with the many possibilities for personal advancement it offers.

Table Of Contents

Introduction

There are numerous sports that are played all around the world by a wide range of people. Ensuring that everyone is in the best health possible and sports related injuries are treated properly has created a huge need for sports medicine. While it may seem almost trivial to devote an entire practice of doctors to sports medicine there are numerous reasons why it is a wise decision to make.

Rather than simply working with doctors who are not widely trained in the specific injuries that can occur from sports related injuries it is possible to work with a sports medicine doctor. These doctors are specially trained in working with athletes to improve strength, as well as help injuries heal quickly and with as few long-term effects as possible.

Many athletes are injured each year, and often by specializing in sports medicine, the highly trained doctors can gather information and ideas about how to help prevent the injuries from occurring as well as how to help the injuries heal as quickly as possible. Working with a typical doctor will almost always result in a healed injury but it can take much longer, and depending upon the type of injury can result in your athletic career being over. The job of a sports medicine doctor is to ensure that through appropriate treatment, strength building, and diagnostics that you are not left sitting on the sidelines.

Advances in modern medicine have made it possible to narrow down how potential injuries can occur. It is a well-known fact that some sports are tougher on the body than others are, however this inability to all doctors to distinguish what the most serious injuries are often leads them to treating the minor injuries first. A sports medicine doctor is trained to focus on the most pressing injuries first and then worry about those that are not as important. This means if you have an injury to your knee that can affect all of your movement as well as walking on a permanent level they are going to focus more time on your knee rather than the sprained ankle you may have as well.

While the idea of sports medicine seems to be solely related to sports and athletes many dancers find relief from sports medicine doctors as well. Because dancing particularly ballet, jazz and modern are not considered sports some are confused about what benefits a sports medicine doctor can offer. However, if you consider that dancing is a very high stress activity that places great amounts of pressure and strain on your body it makes perfect sense to see a sports medicine doctor. Whenever a dancer sustains an injury while doing Pointe work or practicing for a performance, they are almost always referred by the dance master to a sports medicine doctor to help speed the recovery process.

Aside from just being a pricy specialty there are so many benefits to using sports medicine doctors that many athletes simply will not use a standard doctor unless they are forced to. The added knowledge and experience that sports medicine training provides to doctors is almost unmatched in terms of treating injuries both with and without surgical means. Looking beyond the initial injury and treating the overall cause as well as the injury is one of the biggest goals and helping all athletes return to full strength is a much needed benefit.

1. A Short Description Of Sports Medicine

Sports medicine is a relatively new field or subsection of medicine. Although it has solid roots in the past, its existence is very much a part of the history of the 20th and 21st centuries. Sports medicine is a growing field of employment due to the explosive expansion in sports and athletic activities. Not only are there the traditional high school, professional and amateur sports, there are also the "extreme" sports.

With every athletic event, there is risk of injury. In the instances of the so-called extreme versions, the likelihood of accidents and harm to the body increases. The focus of sports medicine is on the proper functioning of the human body during athletics and sporting competitions. Its concern is to prevent and treat any possible injuries resulting from such activities.

There is a demand for practitioners in the discipline of sports medicine. The need for people to be able to diagnose and manage sporting injuries is increasing proportionately to the interest in extreme, elite, professional amateur and recreational sports. Employers vary from professional team owners or managers to elite athletes to high schools and colleges. Anyone interested in pursuing a career in this field of study and work will find him or herself facing an ever-widening choice of possible employment.

The field of sports medicine is growing because it is a varied one. It is not a single sphere of expertise. The term "sports medicine" is a wide umbrella encompassing diverse professions. It is not a single profession. This makes the term hard to define, but it opens up many different doors of employment for now and in the future.

Where specifically does a specialist in sports medicine find work? The specialist works with athletes in the field and in a clinical setting. He or she may become a team physician or an athletic trainer. There are those in sport medicine who practice as orthopedic surgeons, exercise physiologists, biomechanists, physical therapists, sports psychologists and sports nutritionists. All have their own niche within this diverse subsection of medicine.

To become a member of the sports medicine team requires a certain character. At its basic is congeniality and someone with above average people skills. A person interested in becoming involved in most fields of sports medicine must like working with and being in the company of others. Daily interactions may involve meetings with officials, researchers, peers, athletes and family members.

The job also demands the individual possess a specific set of learning skills. An interest in the sciences must go hand-in-hand with a concern in sports. There is also the need for education and, in many instances, more education. A person does not become a sports medicine professional or even a practitioner over night. It takes time, effort and plenty of energy.

The path to becoming a part of the sports medicine world requires dedication and an awareness of what and what not to do to reach the ultimate goal. It is not smooth or simple. It requires the individual to be aware of whom he or she is. Yet, understanding personal character is not enough. To reach the prerequisite level requires the ability to reduce the vast possibilities to a more singular focus.

Along the way, the candidate for a career in sports medicine must carefully hone his and her people and educational skills. A direction must be selected. After doing this, the individual must direct all energy, effort and drive towards achieving the final goal.

This book will not provide all the answers. No book can. The following pages will act, however, as a basic guide on how to get there. It will also provide some essential and informative information on the field of sports medicine. Some will be simple background material; other sections will focus on education and preparing yourself for the purpose of employment in sports medicine.

This book will begin simply. It will start at the beginning of sports medicine. In doing so, it will provide you with a brief look at the history and development of sports medicine over time.

2. A Historical Account Of Sports Medicine

While the history of sports medicine is recent, it does have antecedents that precede the current modern state. In fact, arguments provide evidence for the practice of a form of sports medicine throughout classical times. There are also indications that vestiges of this specific area of medical practice existed in India, China, and Persia and throughout parts of the Middle East. Texts and vestiges of diverse works relating to healthy exercise practices, sports and/or medicine mention the intermeshing aspects of and the possible harmonization the 2 areas.

The Early Years Of Sports Medicine

The *Atharveda* or *Arthar-Veda*, (ca 6,000 B.C.) an early Indian text, contains some 6,000 lines describing specific healing or therapeutic exercises. Yet, it is not India's only claim to an early form of sports medicine. Sushruta (Susruta), an Indian physician, was the first know doctor to prescribe exercises. He worked at the University in Benares around 600 B.C. where he taught medicine and surgery. However, the favored so-called founders of sports medicine are generally noted to be rooted in Classical Greece.

The so-called Father of Sports Medicine is generally believed to have been the Greek, Herodicus of Selymbria (5th century B.C.) A teacher of sports, he began to study medicine. As a result, he developed a theory of the relationship between medical conditions and therapeutic exercises. Unfortunately, his student Hippocrates, the Father of Medicine, did not completely share his beliefs. While there are no documents remaining to support his claim, the fragments quoted by other classical scholars clearly indicate the right of Herodicus to claim this position.

While there are successive and successful Greek claimants with writings linking sports and medicine, e.g. Plato, Socrates, the next individual commanding specific attention is Ikkos of Tarentum (444 B.C.E). He was another Greek with an interest in combining sports and medicine. He was a physical education teacher. He also, in fact, wrote the first known textbook on athletic training. However, it was not until Claudius Galen (131-201 A.D.) that a text coherently combined philosophy, medicine and exercise. He combined the different aspects together in his text, *Thrasybulus*. The material comprising this book was gleaned partially from observation and directly from his work. Galen was responsible for maintaining the health of Roman gladiators. This makes Galen a candidate for being the first team doctor in recorded history. During the centuries that followed, medical authors borrowed heavily from the works of Galen and the Classical Greek and Roman scholars.

Middle Ages And The Renaissance Period

After the decay and fall of the Roman Empire, in the West, little advances were made in the area of medicine, let alone in sports medicine. The Roman Catholic Church had a distinct way of regarding the human body and its workings. However, great advances in medicine in the East were to have an impact on the field. Ibn S'lna, better known as Avicenna (980-1606) developed and wrote on certain healing exercises. Later, Girolamo Mercuriale or Hieronymous Mercuralis (1530-1606) offered his own vision and version of the medical aspects of physical exertion. He recorded them in his 8-volume work *Libri de Arte Gymnastica*.

Modern Sports Medicine

The modern history of sports medicine was a collaborative effort. Countries and individuals worked together and apart to develop the field. In the early 20th century, work in Germany and Switzerland pushed forward the idea of the two different areas of study working together. Van der Berg of Switzerland is touted for his work on cycling and the heart in 1906. Dresden, Germany boasts having several firsts in the early years of the century. These include first sports physician, first laboratory for the evaluation of athletic performers, first sports medicine journal and first sports medicine association. The term "sports medicine" was yet to be promulgated. There was not yet a cohesive comprehension of the ideals and approaches later declared to be integral to the practice of sports medicine. These were to come about in association with the famous sporting event – the Olympics.

In 1920, the Association Internationale Medico-Sportive (Association International of Sports Medicine) or AIMs came into being. This was the same year for the origin of the German Academy for Physical Exercise in
Berlin. The German Association of Physicians for the Promotion of Physical Culture also began a scholarly periodical in 1924. This was the first recorded sports medicine journal.

In 1928, the group decided to hold a conference in Amsterdam, Holland in conjunction with the 9th Summer Olympic Games at St. Moritz, Switzerland. This first conference saw the attendance of some 280 sports physicians representing at least 20 countries. It was here, at the conference, that the term "sport medicine" came into accepted and more common usage. In fact, the conference bore the name of the International Congress of Sports Medicine. One of the most prominent members was Buytendijk of Switzerland.

The year 1930s and 1940s saw several advances made in the world of sports medicine. The AIMS changed its name to the Fèdèration Internationale Medico-Sportive et Scientifique (FIMS) in 1933 at a meeting in Chamoix, France. The Second International Congress took place in 1933 in Turin, Italy. It became the first general text in the United States for Sports Medicine.

In Germany, Dr. F. Hexheimer wrote the first book containing the words "sports medicine" in the title. This was the *Grundriss der Sportsmedizin*. The country also established the first outpatient department for sports medical outpatients in 1947. Meanwhile, in the United States, Dr. Augustus Thorndike of Harvard published his book *Athletic Injuries, Prevention, Diagnosis and Treatment* in 1938. Dr. Jack Houghston established the Houghston Sports Medicine Hospital in 1949. It was the first of its kind in the United States

Sports Medicine After World War II

After the Second World War, the interest in sports Medicine grew. In 1950, a sports medicine department was established at the university in Leipzig. In England, Sir Adolphe Abrahams and Sir Arthur Porritt founded the British Association of Sport and Medicine (BASM). By 1954, the Americans had begun to make their mark in this field of study. It started with the founding of the American College of Sports Medicine (ACSM) in 1954. A Dr. Edward Hitchcock was teaching at Amherst College in 1954, the first instructor of physical education and hygiene. He also became the country's first sports medicine physician when he began to take care of the teams of his college.

By the end of the 1960s, several countries had established organizations focusing on the interconnection between sports and medicine. In 1960, the Jongbloed group had focused on basic research in the sports medicine field while, in 1962, J.P. G. Williams wrote the first English book with the words "Sports Medicine" in the title. It was called *Sports Medicine*. 1963 saw the creation of Sports Medicine Australia (SMA) as well as Sports Medicine New Zealand (SMNZ). An interest in medicine and sport was expressed in a series of articles published as part of a series written by Ernst Franz Jokl (1907-1997) and P. Jokl. Dr. Robert Kerlan joined forces with Dr. Jobe to create the South Western Orthopedic Medical Group. By 1985, this Group had become the Kerlan-Jobe Orthopedic Clinic.

By the end of the decade, a Canadian, Dr. J. C. Kennedy, irrevocably linked sports and medicine together. In 1968, he attended the Summer Olympic Games in Mexico City. He reported his observations on sports, athletic performance and medicine. In 1970, he went on to help found the Canadian Academy of Sports Medicine (CASM). In 1972, he proved the increasing acceptance of sports and medicine as a field of study when he was appointed the position of Chief Medical Officer of the very first acknowledged medical team at the Summer Olympics in Munich, Germany.

The advances in this direction continued throughout the 1970s. The first edition of an American Journal focusing on Sports Medicine was published in the 1970s. It was the child of Jack Hughston. He had been chair of the Committee of Sports Medicine first formed in 1964 as part of the American Academy of Orthopedic Surgeons (AAOS).The Committee evolved into the American Orthopedic Society for Sports Medicine (AAOSSM) by 1975. The AAOSSM quickly emerged as a viable organ for the movement. It took over the responsibility of the newly named *American Journal of Sports Medicine (AJSM)* in 1974 under the advice of Hughston.

Yet, it was not until 1989 that the American Board of Medical Specialties (ABMS) decided to recognize sports medicine as a legitimate subspecialty. Since then, such organizations as the ACSM have grown. Today, it consists of approximately 20,000 chapter members situated in places across the United States and around the globe. It has become one of the largest organizations focusing on sports medicine and the science of exercise. Other organizations and associations have since made sports medicine an expanding filed of integrated interests. In 1981, the Arthroscopy Association of North America came into existence, as did the American Medical Society for Sports Medicine (AMSSM) in 1991.

Important Timelines In Sports Medicine History

- 6,000 B.C. - The *Atharveda* (India)

- 600 B.C. - Sushruta (Susruta), an Indian physician

- 5th century B.C. - Herodicus of Selymbria: Father of Sports Medicine

- 444 B.C.E - Ikkos of Tarentum -

- 131-201 - A.D.Claudius Galen - *Thrasybulus*

- 980-1606 - Ibn S'lna (Avicenna)

- 1530-1606 - Girolamo Mercuriale or Hieronymous Mercuralis - *Libri de Arte Gymnastica*

- 1903 - Van der Berg of Switzerland work on cycling and the heart

- 1920 - the Association Internationale Medico-Sportive (International Association of Sports Medicine) or AIMs

- 1920 – first sports college with a sports medical curriculum in Berlin

- 1924 – the German Association of Physicians for the Promotion of Physical

Culture publishes the first journal on sports medicine

- 1928 – First formal recognition of name at the first conference held by AIMS –The International Congress of Sports Medicine

- 1933 – AIMs renamed the Fèdèration Internationale Medico-Sportive et Scientifique or FIMS

- 1933 founding of American Academy of Orthopedic Surgeons (AAOS).

- 1933 – Second national congress of FIMS

- 1933 – *Grundriss der Sportzmedizin* by Dr. F. Hexheimer contains the words "Sports Medicine" in title

- 1938 - Dr. Augustus Thorndike of Harvard - *Athletic Injuries, Prevention, Diagnosis and Treatment* became standard text for sports medicine

- 1953 – founding of British Association of Sports and Medicine (BASM)

- 1954 - Standing Committee on Sports Injuries formed by the American Medical Association (AMA)

- 1954 – founding of American College of Sports Medicine (ACSM)

- 1959 – The Standing Committee becomes the Committee on the Medical Aspects of Sports

- 1960 – Unesco's International Council of Sport and Physical Education

- 1962 – J. P. Williams publishes first English book with "Sports Medicine" in the title: *Sports Medicine*

- 1963 - Sports Medicine Australia (SMA)

- 1963 – Sports Medicine New Zealand (SMNZ) founded

- 1962 - Committee of Sports Medicine - Jack Hughston, chair

- 1968 - Dr. J. C. Kennedy - Summer Olympic Games in Mexico City

- 1970 – Canadian Academy of Sports Medicine (CASM)

- 1972 Dr. J. C. Kennedy Chief Medical Officer at Summer Olympics in Munich, Germany

- 1973 – Dr. Robert K. Kerlan and Dr. Frank Jobe open the highly acclaimed Kerlan-Jobe Orthopedics Clinics for sports medicine

- 1974 - *American Journal of Sports Medicine (AJSM)*

- 1975 – American Orthopedic Society for Sports Medicine (AOSSM)

- 1989 - the American Board of Medical Specialties (ABMS) recognizes sports medicine as a sub-specialty

- 1992 – National Sports Medicine Institute of the United Kingdom

- 1994 – Sports Science Institute of South Africa

- 1995 – Combined Congress in Hong Kong of International Arthroscopy Association (IAA) and the International Society if the Knee (ISK)

- 1995 - IAA & ISK combine to form the International Arthroscopy, Knee Surgery and Orthopaedic Sports Medicine (ISAKOS)

- 2001 – founding of United Kingdom Association of Doctors in Sport (UKADS)

Chapter Overview

While sports medicine is a recent development in the world of medicine. It is not a new concept. The history of sports medicine is closely allied with the development of medical practices of the ancient worlds of India, China, Persia, Greece and Rome. Many of the early physicians developed an interest in the relationship between athletic performance and medicine. Some focused on exercise and health. Others looked at specific links between health and athleticism.

During the Middle Ages and the Renaissance, developments were restricted. Many physicians built recited or built slightly on earlier findings. It was not until the late 19th century with the resurrection of the Olympic Games that the interest was revived in the interconnection between sports and medicine. Sports medicine began its journey towards acceptance as a medical sub-specialty during the early 20th century. The formation of various national and international organizations helped to increase the interest in the nature and character of this field of study.

Acceptance in 1989 by the American medical professional organization ABMS served to increase the impetus of has since resulted in a blossoming of individuals whose focus is on sports medicine. Today, the field of sports medicine is a burgeoning one. The next chapter will look at how to assess whether you are suitable for entering a career in this field.

3. A Self-Assessment Guide

So, you want to work in sports medicine. Do you have what it takes? Do you know what it is? Are you suitable for a career in the field? These are basic questions you need to consider before you opt for what can be a long road. Becoming involved in sports medicine can be a rewarding career. It can also be time consuming and very demanding. This chapter will look at whether you are the right material – a good match, for a position in sports medicine. It begins with clarifying exactly what sports medicine is.

Type Of Work

Sports medicine is among the newest types of medical practices. It is a subspecialty that focuses on 2 inter-related aspects of modern life – physical exertion and medicine. Physical exertion describes and encompasses exercise, recreation and sports. It embraces the medical knowledge that comes into play on the different levels of a body in motion and exertion during sporting activities. In understanding this, sports medicine also considers the effect of age and even gender-specific aspects of sports.

Female athletes differ physically from male athletes. This includes the changing physiology that stretches over an individual's lifespan. The age of the player of any sport will also affect the way a practitioner or researcher in the field looks at the data and develops recommendations, training schedules and diet. The role of a sports medicine practitioner must vary in comprehension of these different and unique characteristics for gender and age. He or she would not expect to observe the same pattern of injuries in both an adult or mature athlete and a child or adolescent. Older persons also have their age-specific requirements. A sports medicine practitioner must be aware of all this and more.

A sports medicine practitioner is someone who observes the various types of sports and notices the effects of each kind on those who play. A sports medicine practitioner is also an individual who chooses and/or adapts to the player's milieu. In sports medicine, the professional must be ready to treat injuries and/or accidents that occur both on and off the field. The person in this area of medical practice must also be able to demonstrate how proper and even improper sports training can affect all members of the sporting community and the world beyond it.

As a result, being a sports medicine professional offers plenty of opportunities in various medical and medical-related fields. All concentrate on athletic performance, yet all are applicable beyond the scope of the professional sporting person's venue. While sport specific injuries may result in a somewhat narrow focus, the field of sports medicine, itself, is expansive in encompassing a wide variety of medical specialties. Diagnostic and surgical specialists exist in conjunction with athletic trainers. Rehabilitation coexists with field advice while training advice on physical exercise regimes shares the locker room with psychological assessments.

As a result, sports medicine is a multi-faceted discipline. There are many options and diverse routes to follow to become a member of this diverse group of professionals. It is up to the individual to decide what best suits him or her and which area of expertise will prove to be the right calling. However, before he or she embarks upon what can be a rewarding career, it is first necessary to look at the characteristics that are necessary to become a first-rate practitioner in the field of sports medicine.

Character Evaluation

The first question to ask yourself is this: "Do you like working with people?" If the answer is, "No" go no further. Sports medicine professionals work with people on a daily basis. Depending upon the path a person takes, an average day might involve spending all day with several clients or only with 1.

A practitioner may come into regular contact with other people during his or her work. There are the families of athletes as well as patients and professional to meet and deal with on a regular basis. There are also colleagues and other professionals. You may be providing them with support or they may be seeking your expertise. Contrarily, you may be asking a peer for support or an opinion on a specific matter or case. Overall, excellent people skills are a very basic requirement of being a successful sports medicine professional.

Besides a pleasant disposition as part of a professional manner, the candidate for a spot in a sports medicine program must exhibit excellent interpersonal skills. These include:

- **Verbal Communication**
  The ability to talk to people in a straightforward, confident, comprehensive and knowledgeable fashion – to communicate without "dumbing down" or convoluting the matter at hand

- **Written Communication**
  The ability to write clearly and effectively, to communicate what is required to the different personalities involved

- **Conflict management**
  Preventative and proactive ability to mediate between opposing views and needs

- **Sensitivity**
  To the needs of others

- **Ability to listen**
  To be able to actually hear what the other
  person is telling you, not what you think
  they should be telling you or what you
  want to hear

- **Intergroup dynamics**
  Comprehension of the basic workings of
  groups and associations, an awareness of
  how individuals react and interact in a
  group setting

- **A sense of how you fit into the overall
  scheme of the athlete's world**
  Including life goals, training aspirations and
  both future and immediate needs

While you may be able to develop or improve on
your innate personal skills and characteristics, it is
essential you possess the basis – the very core at the
beginning. If you lack them entirely, it would be
better to go into a more solitary field such as
research.

While not essential, it is also helpful if the
individual has drive, energy and motivation. A
sports medicine professional needs to know what
he or she wants. The person must also have the
energy to sustain the desire through the long
course of education and training. Without the drive
and the energy to complete the course (pun

intended), the chances of going forth in the right direction successfully diminish considerably.

Motivation also plays an important role in obtaining the ultimate goal. An individual must really want to become a sports medicine professional. If he or she (or you) do not really want to achieve this result, it will not happen. The world of professional sports is full of motivated people. It is a necessary requirement if they want to become a successful player. The same is true for sports medicine. The motivating force must be strong, consistent and constant. Furthermore, possessing the motivation to become a sports medicine professional will help you understand the forces that compel an athlete to want to achieve at almost any cost.

Personal Interests

While assessing your capabilities to become a sports medicine professional, it is essential you look at all aspects of your life and lifestyle. This includes considering your own personal interests. What do you enjoy doing when you are at home, at school or in a chosen environment? What do you read, play or do in your spare time? Do you have any spare time?

There are certain core interests common to many historical and current sports medicine personalities. Among the most basic are these top 4: study/school favorites, reading materials, activities and volunteering. Your personal preferences or leanings will help indicate whether you are suited towards a career in sports medicine. It is not too early to ask these questions when you are in public school. It is more appropriate to do so, however, when you are ready to start high school.

The process of this type of self-discovery or self-exploration is simple. Ask yourself the following questions:

1. When at school, do you enjoy studying sciences? Are anatomy, studies of the body's needs, biology and physiology among your favorite subjects?

2. When you pick up a magazine, newspaper or book, what do you prefer to read? Do you turn immediately to articles on nutrition, science, sports and fitness? Do your eyes constantly wander from the latest news on the front page to the sports' section of a newspaper? Are your favorite journals or periodicals on sports and/or medical-related topics?

3. When you spend time on the internet what do you do searches on or research? Is it the latest musical trends, idle twitters or something related to sports and the demands it makes on the body?

4. Are you a part of a team or individual sport in school? Are you physically active? Do you enjoy planning an exercise program or trying out 1 from a magazine?

5. Where do you volunteer? Do you spend time at a hospital, a local medical clinic, a gym, a fitness center or an athletic field?

Answer the questions honestly. If you do love science classes, this is a good sign. If you combine this awareness with an interest in how the body works, it is even better. If you can add to this, an attraction to sports, it is a clear indication that a career in sports medicine is a distinct possibility.

Having a healthy curiosity about and interest in sports and the body is an important aspect of this field of study. It is not enough that an individual understands the anatomy and physical workings of the human body. In sports medicine, the person has to comprehend how the body acts during and training for a sporting event. It is also critical there is an insight into how a person involved in sports thinks and feels.

If an individual truly desires to know how an athlete "ticks," the psychological awareness of sporting minds can help. It is critical to be able to consider more than your own point of view. Studying the subject, reading further on the topics helps gain knowledge on the academic level. Playing and volunteering in sports and medical-related fields provides a practical understanding. If the individual is able to add together the 2 related aspects of sports medicine, it will provide a solid basis upon which to build – to expand upon and grow. These are the very essentials the very foundations of what can become a successful career as a sports medicine practitioner.

Initial Educational Requirements

Yet, even if you enjoy working with people, have the right type of personality and lean towards certain related interests, it is also essential to consider your current educational direction. If you do not have the right academic background, it may prevent, or at least slow down your chances to become involved in the sports medicine field. It is necessary to think ahead, to map out your educational strategy. You have to take the right subjects now in order to achieve the requirements for entry in the ideal college or university. You may think the path starts as soon as you start attending college. This is wrong. You need to prepare yourself the instant you step into your classes in high school. You need from the start to pick your courses wisely.

A high school diploma is a necessity these days for obtaining employment or heading on to college. At the high school level, you will need to focus on sciences. It is essential to have math in its many varied forms, but you need to take and shine in the science courses. Any course work focusing on human physiology will help. Most high schools offer classes in health and biology.

To find out what will help you make it to the next level of your goal, make an appointment with your school's guidance counselor. Ask about college requirements. Maybe arrange to take an aptitude test to help confirm your ability to choose an appropriate career path. See if the counselor has any suggestions about course work or can recommend specific colleges.

If you wish to get another opinion, seek out a sports medicine practitioner or visit a sports clinic. A practitioner in either venue can help. Talk to them about their specialty. Discover how they got there and why they opted for this particular field of sports medicine. He or she will be able to provide some insight into what to take and how to go about it. A practitioner may be able to recommend a course of action. He or she can also suggest promising colleges to consider. If it is at all possible, talk to more than 1 sports medicine professional. It will help you gain some perspective on the diverse nature of the field. It may also provide you with guidance in what direction will work best for you.

Planning For Your Direction

It is an important part of managing your goal to know where you want to go. Early in your high school days, stop and compile a list of possible colleges. Talk to your guidance counselor and a sports practitioner. Compare their suggestions then set about doing your own research.

When looking at different schools remember this fact. The college you want to attend and the college you should attend may not be the same. Look at the various possibilities objectively. Focus on the admission requirements. Do not forget the financial cost. Look at financial assistance programs and find out the rate of placement for graduates of the specific programs. Be thorough even if this is an initial foray. Do start early but do not restrict yourself at this initial stage. A better prospect may come to light at a later date and/or after further research. Furthermore, what you find out initially may not be either feasible or fit in with your career focus at a later date.

Chapter Overview

In order to be acceptable and to consider sports medicine a viable career option, the individual has to be able to meet certain requirements. They are as follows:

- Someone with a science background

- An individual who has an interest in sports

- A high school diploma with subjects in science

- A volunteer record in sports clubs and associations

- Time spent helping out in a health-related environment

- A person who enjoys working with people and helping them solve their problems

- An individual who has drive, energy and a clear understanding of who he or she is and where he or she want to go

The next chapter will look at how to take this basic knowledge a step further. It will focus on the different paths to becoming a member of the study and profession of sports medicine. It will examine the different career paths available and the educational possibilities. It will also explore some basic methods on how to realize the ultimate goal.

4. Possible Career Choices

There are many different paths to follow to become a sports medicine professional. It is a complex field not a single entity. Many different types of medical professionals practice or focus on sports medicine. It is, as is often noted, a collection of different specialties or subspecialties and not a single or distinct practice. This makes it sometimes difficult to comprehend. At the same time, it makes it a delightful overabundance of possible career choices. To provide you an idea of what comprises the subspecialty known as sports medicine, simply look at the list of possible categories, a brief typology as it were.

The Diverse Fields To Consider

If you wish to become a professional in sports medicine, it helps to narrow down your area of interest or expertise. To begin the process, consider first a partial list of the disciplines practicing sports medicine and their base of operation.

Athletic Trainer Or Sports Therapist

- Works with the coaches, team physicians and others

- goal is to prevent and treat any sports-related injuries or illnesses

Biomechanic/Kinsiologist

- Works in clinics and in research facilities

- Applies the laws of physics to sports and physical activities

Chiropractor

- May work in a clinical setting, in the field or out of his or her office

- Treats joints and muscles

Exercise Physiologist

- Traditionally worked with athletes, now may be found in a clinical or commercial setting

- Study the physiological responses of the human body to exercise and other forms of physical activity

Fitness Instructor/Personal Trainer

- One-on-one work

- May go to the athlete's home, training facilities or gym

Massage Therapist

- May be found in a fitness or spa facility

- Tends to be one-on-one but can be hired for a team

Nutritionist/Sports Dietician

- May work in a clinic, do research or perform on an individual consulting basis

- Relieve muscle pain, spasms, tension, fluid retention and other related physical problems

Occupational Therapist

- Works in sports clinics or as consultants to professional sports organizations

- Focuses on the development of motor skills and dexterity

Orthopedist

- Often a specialty field within this musculoskeletal specialty

- Diagnoses and treats bone disorders and diseases

- Can work with a team or become an orthopedic surgeon

Physical Therapist

- Provide evaluation and treatment of injuries

- Relieve pain and increase mobility

- Often concerned with rehabilitation regimes

- Work in sports clinics or as consultants to professional sports organizations

Podiatrist

- Focus is on the foot, ankle and other related parts

- Work in hospitals, private offices and clinics

Researcher In Exercise Scientist

- Usually found in research facilities

- Conducts studies using either a clinical or basic approach

Sports Medicine Physician/Medical Doctor

- Employed by teams but may also work in sports clinics

- Trained to diagnose and treat sport-related injuries

Sports Psychologist

- May work out of a home office or a clinic

- May be in the employ of an individual athlete or a team

- Focuses on the aspects of maintaining and achieving optimal mental health

Strength And Conditioning Coach

- Work for athletic teams at all levels

- Intent is to enhance performance through developing training plans

The Major Areas Of Specialization

If you plan to become involved in sports medicine, a simple way of looking at the various options is this. Divide them into specific categories according to their approach or their focus. You can also analyze them in relation to the type of education they will require. Another method to simplify the various types is to consider the aspect of their focus – sports or science, applied research, fieldwork, or laboratory research. Below is one way of considering the various areas of specialization.

1. **Coaching/training**
   An active and practical application of the principles of sports medicine

2. **Science of Exercise**
   Focusing on the physical can be academic or practical in nature and/or application

3. **Physical And Athletic Training**
   Hands-on work involving athletes. Field
   and clinical work

4. **The Promotion Of Physical Health And Fitness**
   A practical approach of academic subjects
   directed towards a larger audience or
   restricted to the select few clients

Educational Qualifications For Each Field

Educational requirements to enter university are
specific. To become involved in the world of sports
medicine, however, requires paying rigorous
attention to detail. The intensity of the educational
qualifications depends entirely upon the direction
the individual decides to take. If you decide to
become a sports doctor, be prepared to go beyond
university to take a medical degree, an internship
and even a specialized residency. At the very
minimum, someone in the sports medicine field
will require an academic degree in an accredited
institution.

Your future does rely on you selecting the right
university. You need to investigate the various
college options available to you. Do your research
on the internet, but also talk with actual persons
involved in the field. This chapter will consider
more of the process of getting into the right college
and graduate studies in the next section. This

portion of the chapter is focusing on the different routes for the different types of sports medicine.

You need to study the coursework offered by the college or university. The basic coursework for a sports medicine degree program should include sciences with a concentration on the mechanism of the human body. A general degree would include such things as psychology, nutrition, a history of sports and basic anatomy. A Bachelor of Science (BSc) is a basic requirement. The focus should be on applied health sciences as well as exercise science, adult fitness and general sports.

Those involved in furthering their education will also be considering such things as courses in such specific and more advanced courses as orthopedics, therapy, chiropractic applications, musculoskeletal injuries, genetics and sports-related or sports-specific injuries.

It is necessary to be completely aware of the basic criteria and/or educational requirements for each type of sports medicine. Some, such as Massage Therapist require completion and certification through a training program. Others demand at least a 4 or 5-year degree from an accredited college or university. These include Athletic Trainers, Fitness Instructors, Exercise Physiologists, and Physical Therapists. Nutritionists need an undergraduate degree followed by an internship while Occupational Therapists need an undergraduate degree and specialized coursework. Biomechanics specialists must have a Masters degree as do those who plan to be Strength and Conditioning Coaches. A PhD is the basic requirement of a chiropractor and for a researcher in Exercise Science. If you want to be an orthopedist, a podiatrist or a sports medicine doctor, you must finish medical school and do an internship. These fields also require taking coursework and doing practicum work in the areas of specialization.

Educational Planning For Career Pathing

When you do decide to go to university, plan far ahead. Give yourself plenty of opportunity and time to make the decision on the right school for your career. You will need to research thoroughly. There are several reasons for this. While many schools may offer courses on science or physiology, not all are related to or applicable to sports medicine.

Furthermore, certain types of sports medicine occupations are sticklers for where you obtain your degree or certificate. If you want to become an Athletic Trainer, you need to graduate from a college program approved by the Commission on Accreditation of Allied Education Programs. If you plan to become a Sports Dietician or Nutritionist, you need your degree and a 9-month internship approved by the American Dietetics Association (ADS). The National Strength and Conditioning Association (NSCA) recommend that all Strength and Training Coaches take part in the Certified Strength and Conditioning Specialist Program.

It is not difficult to find out what colleges, courses and universities are accredited and/or preferred. Talk to a guidance counsel, go on line and read the information provided on sports medicine careers. Read the American College of Sports Medicine's (ACSM) directories. There is a graduate and undergraduate directory for you to consult.

All recommended sites and literature generally provide basic information on the educational requirements. Some go further. They provide a list of colleges to examine and specific descriptions of requirements and coursework. Some sites even provide you with links to associations and organizations.

Some organizations to consider in North America are the following:

- The American College of Sports Medicine

- The American Osteopathic Academy of Sports Medicine

- The American Academy of Podiatric Sports Medicine

- The American Orthopedic Society for Sports Medicine

- The Canadian Academy of Sports Medicine

- The Institute for Preventive Sports Medicine

- The American Massage Therapy Association

- The American Academy of Physical Medicine and Rehabilitation

- The International Society of Biomechanics in Sport

- The National Strength and Conditioning Association

- World Council on Orthopaedic Sports Medicine

Doing online research is not enough. It is also not sufficient to speak only to a counselor, however, well informed he or she may be. Make sure you do speak to someone in the field. Go to a sports clinic or talk to a coach. Speak to a member of the specific association on line. They can help clarify the educational expectations of their organization and area of expertise. If you have any questions, do not hesitate to ask them. It is better you do so at the beginning before it is too late.

An excellent way to narrow down your choice is to visit the campus. See if there is an open house or prospective student day or week. If you go to the campus, you can connect with the different elements that will make the learning experience work in your favor. Talk to present students and faculty if possible. Sit in on a class. Collect any information and add it to your definite, maybe or "no way ever" list.

If you are uncertain about what fields to take or what direction to head in, consider "shadowing." Try to locate someone in any of the interested areas of sports medicine. Contact him or her. Ask if it is possible for you to arrange to be with him or her for a workday. This will give you a glimpse into what the work entails. In this way, you can decide for or against entering this particular field of sports medicine.

Shadowing a professional in the sports medicine field of your choice is beneficial in another way. It may provide you with a possible volunteer option or even part-time job. It is very important for you to add to your working knowledge. Education in school is important. Actual work or volunteer experience is as important. In fact, it will create a better impression and add depth to a *curriculum vita*.

If you want to volunteer or add to your status, there are a few approaches to take. You can adopt this approach while you are still in high school. You can carry them over into your college years. Take classes in first aid. Obtain your certificates from St. John's Ambulance, the Red Cross or an equivalent or similar organization. Take your knowledge and volunteer with the school's sports team. You do not have to be an athlete to become involved in sports activities.

Another method of improving your knowledge of sports medicine both before and during college is to attend seminars. Check in your area and see if there are any symposiums, conferences or seminars on sports medicine related topics. Sports Medicine groups post conferences and other gatherings online. Check the schedule and find out if you can attend. If it is restricted, perhaps you can volunteer to work at the symposium. This way you can attend. In some instances, you may even be employed to work the event, thus doubly benefitting from the experience.

The same type of benefits can accrue if you work for a newspaper. It will improve your writing. At university, the chance may expand to submit work for scholarly journals. Some schools publish their own scientific journals. Admittedly, most scholarly periodicals do not publish work from students in the lower levels. You can, however, offer to work with and research for a professor who is doing an article or study for a scholarly journal. By doing so, you may be able to obtain credit in the article as well as name recognition for when you actually submit an article. Below is a list of potential sports medicine journals. Several of them are located in North America while others are found in other countries around the world:

- *The British Journal of Sports Medicine -* Australia

- *The Clinical Journal of Sports Medicine –* Canada

- *The International Journal of Sports Medicine –* Germany

- *The Journal of Athletic Training –* United States

- *Journal of Orthopaedic and Sports Physical Therapy –* United States

- *Journal of Science and Medicine in Sport –* South Australia

- *Journal of Sports Medicine and Physical Fitness* – The Netherlands

- *Journal of Sports Science and Medicine –* Turkey

- *Medicine and Science in Sports and Exercise –* United States

- *Physical Therapy in Sport –* United Kingdom

- *The Physician and Sportsmedicine –* United States

- *Research in Sports Medicine: An International Journal –* Hong Kong

- *Sports Medicine* – United States

- *Sports Medicine and Arthroscopy Review* – United States

Working with and/or for a professor can be beneficial in other ways. It will gain you experience in a specific filed relating to sports medicine. It should also gain you the support of your professor. This will come in handy when you need recommendations for higher learning or are out seeking employment. Your former professor or teacher can provide you with a glowing reference. This will add to the impression you are truly dedicated to and interested in working in the field of sports medicine.

Practical Tips For Career Planning

People are always looking for ways in which they can have a highly successful career and there are things that you can do to really increase the chances of being successful. However, if you simply overlook some tips you can still have a fulfilling career while other tips are quite necessary in order to succeed. Working towards a successful career often begins long before you actually start the career, and sports medicine is certainly no exception.

One of the first considerations that you should look into is ensuring if you are still in school that you are studying enough science to satisfy the needs of sports medicine. If you are someone, who hates biology class, and tries to figure out ways to avoid other science classes then sports medicine may not be the best idea for you. While sports medicine is not always about treating patients, it is still considered a medical field and someone who dislikes science is not likely to find happiness in the field. However, if you really do want to find a career in sports medicine you need to look into taking as much biology, an anatomy and physics class as your school possibly offers.

If you are not in school currently, look for a school that will offer excellent programs in the science fields that are required. If you have already completed your schooling, look and see if your classes that you studied will fulfill the science needs for getting started. If it does not, then it is best to start looking for a school that can satisfy your needs.

Another thing that you should closely look into is selecting the medical school you want to attend. Not all schools are created equally. Students who attend the best schools tend to get a higher quality education and are able to translate that higher education into better careers ultimately. You may have to compare prices of schools to find one you can actually afford, but attending the best school you can possibly afford will certainly pay off in the long run.

While you are looking for the perfect school to attend, consider which area of sports medicine you are interested in specializing in. Most doctors simply cannot attend to all of the medical needs of athletes; there are far too many specialties to even try so it is best that you look for a school that is excellent in your desired specialty. For example, a school that is highly regarded for their training of traditional medical doctors may not be as useful to you if you are looking into a career in orthopedics or even surgery. Ensure you are training for the correct field that you are really interested in.

Look for a residency program that is based in the exact specialty of sports medicine that you are interested in as soon as possible. While all doctors must do basic residency programs, many move on immediately from the residency program into sports medicine. This is not recommended at all, due to the complex nature of the body and the strains as well as considerations when sports are involved it is best to participate in a sports medicine residency program as well before fully starting in the field. This will allow you to maximize your hands on training and get the absolute most possible from all of your education. A career in medicine is certainly not cheap, so do your best to ensure you are putting that education to maximum usage.

Additionally, networking can be your best friend, especially for those who are beginning. Whether you offer your services to a semi professional team, or only to the little league team down the road it gives you the opportunity to help people learn who you are and what you are capable of doing. You simply cannot purchase advertising that is as good for your practice. So volunteer some of your time monitoring games and helping ensure that athletes are taken care of; people will recognize your efforts and are much more likely to use you when they need a sports medicine doctor.

Chapter Overview

The vast variety of possible field in sports medicine makes it critical to carefully select the right course and the right university. Be thorough in your research. Explore all possible venues. Make sure the school is accredited and accepted by your specific sports medicine association or organization.

Talk to current and past students. Speak not once but several times to a guidance council. Make sure your options are clear. Contact the right sports associations. Go online and research, research, research. Make sure this university or college is right for you and acceptable to the field of sports medicine.

Before and during your schooling – both high school and college, do all that you can to prepare yourself for your chosen career in sports medicine. At the same time, do the extra work. Go that extra mile that will clearly set you apart from other candidates to this university and other levels of higher education as well as for future employers. Shadow someone working as a sports medicine practitioner. Take courses in first aid from recognized organizations. Volunteer to help-out with the athletic programs in some fashion. You do not have to play to be a team player.

Go to any extracurricular activities relating to your area of interest. This may be a symposium of specialists in the field. It could be a special seminar or a small regional or larger national conference. Do whatever it takes to develop your skills and indicate to others your interest and dedication to the field of sports medicine.

The next chapter looks at the job market. It will consider the various sources of employment, the available opportunities and provide several hints on how to land a job in sports medicine.

5. Career Breaks

You have made it. You have survived the grueling years in school. You may have even gone to graduate school and ventured further into an internship. Whatever your path, however long it took, you are now officially completed the formal aspect of your education and training. Now, what? Do you have any idea – a remote clue, of where to go or what to do.

The immediate answer to this question is "Find a job." This chapter will look at the various jobs available in your career. It will provide suggestions on where to look. It will also offer various suggestions on how to land a job.

Job Availability

The field of sports medicine has several advantages over other careers and forms of employment. In choosing sports medicine as your career goal, you have given yourself the opportunity to decide where and how you want to work. This is because sports medicine provides its practitioners with choice. Professionals working in sports medicine have a choice of venue as well as setting. A sports person can work alone or with groups. He or she can choose to work either inside or outside. While much depends upon the specific type of sports medicine, there is still plenty of maneuverability and choice with the professions comprising this field of study.

There are 3 basic types comprising the essential character of sports medicine. They focus on the environment or venue of the work pattern. It is the simplest way to divide sports medicine within the broader scope of descriptive and highly volatile contents. It is too difficult to attempt to separate the broader scope along medical and medically-related lines. The most simple and effective way to look at the typology is to consider the basic work settings. In sports medicine, there are 3 basic types of work environment. These are the areas of research/theory, fieldwork and clinical applications.

Research

Research refers to those practitioners who prefer to work in classrooms or laboratories on the theoretical or potential practical application of sports medicine. These professionals focus on what is now and what may be possible.

In sports medicine, laboratory research is an essential part of finding better ways to ensure the body heals faster, moves more efficiently and comes to harm less frequently and with fewer consequences. Those who choose to work in laboratory settings have contact with peers, may work with animals, conduct experiments and prepare reports.

Theoretical applications of sports medicine may refer to those who remain in the laboratories. It can also refer to those who decide to teach. In high schools, universities and colleges across the United States and around the world, there are those who specialize in the theory of sports medicine. They help others learn what sports medicine is and how it applies to the modern world. These professionals must deal with their peers, students and parents. They may also be involved in the local sports teams and in sports medicine advances in the laboratory.

Fieldwork

Fieldwork can be the opposite of research. While it is true, some types of research require field trials, much goes on in the laboratory. Fieldwork, in this instance, refers to those who work with athletes on their own turf, or rink, or gym. A sports medicine professional may decide this is the milieu for him or her. He or she may prefer to apply his or her craft where the athletes are.

Someone who chooses to work in this environment will need to be prepared to deal on a regular basis with athletes, their coaches, managers and support groups. Owners, team managers, families   and the media may all be environmental factors.

Clinical Work

Clinical work can combine fieldwork and research and, even, teaching. This type of sports medicine may also be strictly dealing with clients within the confines of a hospital, clinic or medical office. The practice could consist of the same clients on a regular or irregular basis. It may involve rehabilitation work or nutritional advice.

Working in this type of setting brings the sports medicine professional in contact with a wide range of different people. Some of the daily contacts are others in the sports medicine business. Some are nurses, other doctors and specialists. There are also office support staff and the others who comprise the staffing demands of the average clinic. Someone in a clinical environment has patients who are athletes and those who may be in sport but are not pros or amateurs. Depending upon their status and situation, there are the individual's support staff, including manager, coach and family members.

Sports medicine is different from many other types of jobs or careers. While some of the jobs may be more limited in scope than others, many of the careers in sports medicine allow the practitioner to choose among the different settings. An Aerobics or group instructor may not find him or herself conducting classes in clinical trials or labs. Yet, the instructor may be able to choose whether to teach in clinics, hospitals, schools or industrial settings.

He or she may be private or public. Not many careers offer so many choices.

Basic Jobs

The basic environment for those who practice sports medicine is the clinic, the lab or the field. The setting also indicates the possible employers of those in the profession. The following list consists of the more prominent or common categories of employers of employers in the field of sports medicine:

Professional Sports

The most prominent employer of sports medicine practitioners and the best known is the field of professional sports and its athletes. In this surrounding, the sports medicine professional may supply a number of services. He or she may be an employee of an athlete, a coach, a manager or a team owner. The employer may also be a committee such as the Olympic committee or that in charge of a specific athletic event.

The environment may be a clinic, a locker room, an office or a playing field. It can also be a combination of all of the above. It depends upon the terms of the employment, the specific needs of the athlete or employer and the type of sports medicine practiced or practices. For example, a dietician or sports psychologist may or may not make "field calls.

Amateur Sports

Amateur sports are another large employer of practitioners of sports medicine. These include colleges, universities and high schools. These institutions may hire different types of sports medicine professionals. While some may restrict their involvement to the teams of the schools, others will also act as teachers, counselors, coaches and/or other related positions in this environment.

Jobs In Government

The government hires sports medicine professionals at different levels. These may be for educational purposes. It can involve research facilities. There are specific committees and organizations within the government that may require the expertise of sports medicine professionals.

Clinics

There are various sports medicine clinics across the United States, North America and the world. There are also clinics that include a practitioner of sports medicine on the staff. Clinics devoted to sports medicine provide may also have part-time positions or offer office and/or research privileges.

Other Fields For Practice

It is impossible not to repeat this maxim. Sports Medicine is an area of employment in which there is a multiplicity of different types of employment. While all vary in intensity and direction, all are focused on ensuring quality care in the field of sports medicine. Below is a list and brief description of the most common positions in sports medicine as well as the possible employers and/or work environment. Understanding this will help you understand where to look for employment. It will narrow down the best possibilities.

- Aerobics Instructor - spas, clinics, hospitals, institutions, gyms

- Athletic Trainer – Amateur and professional sports teams, individual athletes

- Biomechanic – research settings, clinical sites

- Chiropractor – clinics, private office or facilities, hospital setting

- Exercise Physiologist – clinics, athletes, commercial settings

- Fitness instructor/Personal Trainer – individual athletes, groups, gyms

- Massage Therapist – sports rehabilitation centers, hospitals, clinics, fitness centers, spas, individuals

- Nutritionist/Sports Dietician – universities, schools, athletes, clinics, hospitals, sports complexes, public health organizations

- Occupational Therapist – hospitals and clinics

- Orthopedist – clinics, hospitals

- Physical Therapist – hospitals, clinics, private offices

- Podiatrist – clinics, hospitals, private office

- Sports Psychologist – research, clinics, teams, sports complexes

- Strength and Conditioning Coach – teams – high school, college, university, professional

There is another reason for keeping in contact with the various associations. They can help you when it comes time to establishing your career. In order to practice in some of the fields of sports medicine, you need to have approval, certification or licenses. These associations are frequently responsible for the granting of the license. These associations may set the test. If this is a matter of state or national business, the association can best inform you of the rules and obligations of your craft for each state.

Some Helpful Advice For The Sports Medicine Job Hunter

Once you decide on where to look for the jobs and know the possible employers, it can facilitate matters. You need to draw up a contact list. You also need to be systematic in your job search. Do not proceed in a haphazard matter. Do keep records of your job search.

While you may be planning on a career in sports medicine, at its basics, the job search process is not different from that for any job. You need to apply yourself in a regular and logical fashion. You need to compile lists. Most important of all – you need to have thought out the plan, established contacts and made the very basics movements towards obtaining employment long before you have graduated.

During your years at school, you need to have done the following to make the job search easier:

- Joined or established connections with a number of organizations or associations in the field of your choice. Write them letters and submit articles to their publications. Make sure you are on the e-mail or mailing list of any or all of the following: The American College of Sports Medicine (ACSM), the American Osteopathic Academy of Sports Medicine (AOADM), the American Academy of Podiatric Sports

Medicine (AAPSM), the Institute for Preventative Sports Medicine (IPSM), the International Association of Arthroscopy, Knee Surgery and Orthopedic Sports Medicine (IAAKSOSM), the International Federation of Sports Medicine (IFSM) and the Canadian Academy of Sports Medicine (CASM). There is also the National Strength and Conditioning Association (NSCA), the Association for the Advancement of Applied Sports Psychology (AAASP) and the American Dietetics Association (ADA)

- Know the local journals – see Chapter 4 and try to be published

- Talk to your professors and instructors. Ask them for suggestions. Make contacts through them

- Put together a professional resume or CV

- Gain and list any and all work experience before after and during your tenure at school

- Be sure you establish a history of volunteerism in the right areas and maintain this while you are in school and applying for jobs. These can be very good contacts

- You are in sports medicine so do not forget to talk to and establish a relationship with the local clubs and sports association

- Talk up yourself to the local pool of athletes and volunteer at local sporting events to show what you are capable of doing

- Know who best to approach to establish your self

- If you are thinking about going it alone, have a solid business plan to present to the possible financers.

- If you want to set up a clinic, talk to like-minded classmates and others in the sports program. This will permit you to spread the financing across many and provide a variety of services under a single roof

Searching for a job – any job, is about contacts. It is about whom you know and whom they may know. It is also about your education. It is about the marks you make - the type of school record that extends beyond the obvious educational aspects of learning.

Yet, job searches are also about hard work. You need to apply yourself. If you do not, nothing will happen. Check posted listings on the internet and in person. Look for openings listed in the periodicals and on the sites of the various associations. Phone, write, e-mail and apply.

Make sure you become members of various list services and internet groups. Yahoo, MSN and others can provide you with certain tools to ensure you make contacts with others.

Chapter Overview

Finding a job in sports medicine is not a given. If you do not go out and use everything you have, you will probably not obtain a job, let alone the job of your dreams. You need to have established a list of potential jobs and a definite list of contacts long before you have graduated. You need to know about licenses and other state or national requirements.

If you not only talk to prospective clients and employers but also listen to professors, teachers, employers, and other sources, you should gain more than a book education during you time spent at school.

6. A Few Issues In Sports Medicine

As add-on trivia, this chapter will focus on current issues involving the practice of modern sports medicine. As you are looking into the possibility of entering this medical field, it is always practical advice to keep abreast with current events and research and development to go in conjunction with your acquired educational qualifications.

Sports Medicine Ventures Into Magnetic Therapy

As research all around the medical field continues to expand, the number of doctors who are looking closely at magnetic therapy continues to grow as well. With side ranges of benefits that can help those in pain without the use of medications, heat or ice this is starting to look like one of the best treatment options available to athletes regardless of the injury. While not everyone is suited to use magnetic therapy, those who have tried it so far have been highly successful and enjoyed the quick results.

Physicians in all medical fields have been studying the effects of magnets on pain, and now the sports medicine field is paying especially close attention. When studying how something can change the healing process sports medicine professionals are always looking at the athlete's health first. Using magnets instead of medications has several benefits including the fact that there are no drugs used when treating injuries with magnets. This reduces the risk of detrimental side effects and also helps to ensure that the athlete is fully alert, rather than groggy from taking pain medications.

It is important however to note that the magnets that medical development is using, is not the standard magnet that you find on your refrigerator. Instead, medical technology is developing biomagnets that are much more effective, and offer the maximum benefits. In addition to treating simple sore areas from injuries, magnets are being used in research to determine their ability to help ease the symptoms of carpal tunnel syndrome as well. The potential benefits to pain treatment are incredible.

Through the continued research into magnets as well as sports medicine fields it seems that the use of magnets is highly anticipated. Doctors have suggested that using the appropriate magnet can reduce healing time for many injuries by as much as half. These types of results are simply phenomenal in a field where quick recovery can mean the difference between a sports career, and sitting on the sidelines watching.

At this time, the number of doctors actively involved in the research of biomagnets if relatively small, however with growing numbers appearing it is a trend that is expected to grow even more in the coming months and years. Many are hoping that the use of the biomagnets will replace all standard heat and ice treatments that athletes are forced to use currently to help speed healing to injuries. While the use of magnets at this point is highly limited, there are many who are carefully watching developments for encouraging signs.

Regardless of sport, magnetic therapy has proven to be a highly effective and versatile treatment option that doctors have to use. With magnets used in various methods, including bracelets and wraps there is almost no limit to the type of injury that is expected to be treatable using magnetic therapy. Sports medicine doctors particularly are looking at the research as highly encouraging because of the vast amount of injuries that they see yearly.

In the meantime, while research continues unfortunately most athletes are forced to continue using the methods of heat and ice to help promote faster healing for their injuries. Once the research is developed further, we can expect that it will be widely available to all athletes, as well as non-athletes alike. From start to finish, magnetic therapy has offered a peek at a much easier and smoother treatment option and while research continues to suggest it is right around the corner there are many who are anxiously awaiting.

For those who are able to see benefits of magnetic therapy now, the results are amazing and provide immediately lower pain levels regardless of whether the pain is from the knee, neck, arm, back, shoulder, or anywhere else. Using the small magnets is a wave from the future and the sports medicine field is anxiously awaiting to see what other great developments are unraveled as the research continues into this important pain relief treatment.

Steroid Use In Sports Medicine

There are always athletes who feel the need to use steroids while playing sports. While many organizations prohibit the usage, the doctors in the sports medicine field tend to be the real people who are fighting the effects of steroids on a daily basis.

Some of the most prevalent symptoms that sports medicine doctors are forced to deal with include mood swings, violent behavior, depression, and psychoses. The good news is that all of these symptoms are reversible with treatment once the use of the steroids stops; however some other conditions are not as easily reversed.

The use of steroids can alter numerous systems in the body, and how they react in terms of permanent or temporary is very important in terms of working to treat the effects. As the number of athletes guilty of using steroids is steadily decreasing there are fewer problems that doctors are trying to counter, however the use of steroids is still happening which causes the problems to still persist even if at a slower level.

While sports medicine doctors do not typically treat reproductive issues, they are finding themselves engaged in more aspects as the use of steroids can hinder several components. For example, in men it can alter the libido, as well as cause male pattern baldness and even cause impaired spermatogenesis amongst the other problems that include testicular atrophy and gynecomastia. However, of all of the problems, only male pattern baldness is entirely non-reversible with treatment. However, there are times when even gynecomastia is unable to be successfully treated once steroid use has been discontinued.

Women tend to have greater reproductive problems with the use of steroids with the risks causing problems with menstrual cycles, an altered libido, deepened voice, pattern baldness, and even clitoral enlargement. The good news is that the libido as well as menstrual cycle can be restored, while the other results of steroid use at this point are not a reversible complication. This means that each year, women who stop taking steroids are still left with the results to deal with, much more so than men are.

Steroids also have the unfortunate problem of negatively affecting the cardiovascular system, which is bad in athletes as they need to be as healthy as possible in order to achieve the best results. With increased LDL cholesterol levels, reduced HDL cholesterol levels, as well as complications with hypertension, elevated triglycerides and even the potential of arteriosclerotic heart disease the use of steroids has several devastating effects on the athletes overall health.

While there are rare and few doctors who will encourage the use of steroids, a well trained doctor will be able to identify signs that an athlete is using steroids and will do their best to help discourage their usage. While obviously the final choice on using steroids lies with the athlete, a good sports medicine doctor should be able to identify based on signs, which athletes are using.

Because of the risks associated with the cardiovascular system as well as musculoskeletal system, using steroids can actually cause more harm to the body than it can provide in benefits. In addition to the complications associated with the cardiovascular system that were already discussed, it can create complications with tendon degeneration, which is potentially not reversible.

This creates a huge problem with weakened tendons that are much more susceptible to injury even after steroid use has stopped. Overall, steroid use represents a huge problem to sports medicine doctors all around the world.

The Purpose Of The American College Of Sports Medicine

The American College of Sports Medicine is more than just a nifty name; they are the main organization that is working towards improving the entire field of sports medicine with the overall health of athletes in mind. By taking the ideas and advances in sports medicine and combining them together with the best training and developmental research, the American College of Sports Medicine aims to help as many people as possible regardless of location.

Developed in 1954, the ACSM has more than 20,000 members currently amongst its ranks with members coming from all around the world. The American College of Sports Medicine is working in several ways to help improve the overall treatment options that are available to athletes around the world, including the use of their certification programs that range from the type of specialty. It is always recommended to select a sports medicine professional who is certified in the area in which they practice to ensure they have received the best training possible.

In addition to the certification programs that are offered the ACSM offers several conferences through out the year in various locations that are geared towards specific specialties. Professionals who are associated with the ACSM are highly encouraged to attend these conferences to help them stay up to date on the latest developments in the field of sports medicine.

In addition to working with professionals who are already practicing a specialty in the sports medicine field, the ACSM also encourages students who are still in school and those involved in their residency to start getting involved to ensure they are expanding their education as much as possible. While some may think that the ACSM is useless, many also agree that there are numerous benefits of having a specific group responsible for giving the certifications.

Most patients prefer working with doctors who are well qualified, and the American College of Sports Medicine offers numerous benefits because of the continued research in the field as well as extensive developmental opportunities that it offers. In addition, the ACSM is dedicated to helping professionals develop as much as possible simply by making it convenient, with a mixture of campus and online programs offered there is almost no reason why every sports medicine professional cannot be involved in continuing their educational goals.

Athletes themselves find the ACSM to be a great resource to them. It provides them a way of measuring various sports medicine professionals to help them determine which the best provider for their individual needs is. By ensuring that a certification method is in place, it allows most athletes and coaches alike to separate the dedicated sports medicine providers from those who are not as experienced and knowledgeable in the field.

As each individual provider grows and expands their knowledge of the field, they are usually welcomed to join the ACSM and ensure that they continue to stay at the top of their field. Various methods are always in place for most fields to keep professionals well trained and the ACSM provides this for the sports medicine field. Despite continuous improvements in treatment options available, the American College of Sports Medicine encourages professionals to continue to be the best in their field.

However, important to note is that aside from the ACSM encouraging doctors and other sports medicine professionals to continuously further their education it also encourages advances in the field to help new treatment methods develop faster, as well as helping ensure that all treatment methods have the best interests of the athletes in mind whom they are designed to help.

Further helping the ACSM is the fact that there are so many resources that are used to help ensure that certified professionals in the sports medicine field stay up to date on all pressing technology changes and new developments. Rather than allowing, all of the professionals to allow their education to take a backseat to their practice professionals are highly encouraged to continue learning as much as possible.

Conclusion

The field of sports medicine is vibrant. It is one offering both opportunity and choice. Sports medicine is not a single entity, a lone profession or a solitary subspecialty. Sports medicine is full of variety. It is an umbrella providing a single name for a group with vastly different and/or wide-ranging skills.

If you want to become a sports medicine practitioner, you have to be gregarious. You need to be a good listener. You also must be self-aware of your potential and capabilities. Decide where you want to go, what you want to take and how to accomplish this before you leave high school.

You need to set the pace of your studies to include volunteering at the right kind of events and activities. You need also to establish a solid working relationship with your teachers/instructors. They may provide work possibilities and suggestions as where to apply for employment after graduation. They can indicate the organizations, associations and periodicals that could be helpful. They can even know about the trends within the field and the best directions to reach your goal. Plan well in advance but be adaptable. If you drive yourself in the right direction, you may be able to score the winning goal, the touchdown, and the perfect score.

As sports medicine has developed over the years, the ideas of how to study and analyze both the athletes and their injuries have increased as well. As time progresses even further, this study is increased as new advances in medicine, training methods and even treatment options are further explored. What seems like science fiction now can very well become a real treatment in the future.

The Future Of Sports Medicine

The idea of sports medicine is very unlikely to waiver. The primary reason being sports are such an integral part of life that most people simply cannot imagine their lives without them. This creates the need to continuously improve upon treatment options for injuries, and also leads to even further research and development required to help reduce the number of injuries that are experienced. While many forms of medicine are simply studying the treatment options heavily, and relying less on preventing problems sports medicine is focused on the long term commitment to athletes by reducing the risks of injury overall through proper training and fitness.

Continuously working to improve fitness and training techniques has ensured that regardless of the treatment options offered, sports medicine has secured itself a very safe home in the medical field. With thousands of new athletes each year starting sports there are always new injuries, as well as new considerations to take into account. These differences can often be a huge aspect when compared to the age of the athlete. Children tend to have more injuries at times, which are due to underdeveloped bones and muscles, while adults tend to have more serious injuries and take much longer to fully heal.

Combining all of the current research with the developments in surgery, fitness, and dietary fields allows sports medicine to continue to grow and encompass the majority of the athlete's life. The desire to play sports for many is not simply a hobby, so selecting a doctor that views it as merely a hobby is unwise. Doctors in the sports medicine field are usually highly dedicated to their work. Putting forth diligent effort to reduce the amount of time to treat injuries, and helping improve the body following an injury are all continuous processes that undergo essential development.

Some of the biggest breakthroughs of recent sports medicine will eventually be classified as obsolete and new, exciting techniques and principals will replace them. Deciding how to carefully advance the research is in the hands of the well-trained doctors who have made it their life's work to help each and every athlete improve their overall health and fitness levels.

From studying exercises to make small adjustments for a positive impact on the entire body, to making slight changes in the way surgery is performed to allow faster recovery times, to even increasing the effort put forth to ensure all athletes are following a healthy diet there is plenty of room for improvements and advances.

In addition to studying the body of the athlete themselves, sports medicine is starting to encompass the rules and structure of games themselves. For example, after a recent study of softball it was determined that breakaway bases should be used to help protect the players. This one small change was estimated to help reduce athlete injuries by as much as 90%. As you can see, sports medicine is encompassing so much more than simply traditional medical aspects as it moves towards the future.

Looking to get your hand on more great books?

Come visit us on the web and check out our great collection of books covering all categories and topics. We have something for everyone.

http://www.kmspublishing.com

Made in the USA
Lexington, KY
31 July 2013